BEYOND TREATMENT

Discover how to build a cellular

foundation to achieve optimal health

John Young, M.D.

Beyond Treatment

Printed in the United States by
Mira Digital Publishing
Chesterfield, Missouri 63005

"The doctor of the future will no longer treat the human frame with drugs, but rather will cure and prevent disease with Nutrition."

Thomas Edison

CONTENTS

Section 2

The Solution: Rebuild your Health at the Cellular Level

Section 3

Client Testimonials

Foreword

by

Professor Michael F. Holick, Ph.D., M.D.

Beyond Treatment provides a refreshing new approach to health and wellness. The adage "You are what you eat" comes across loud and clear in Dr. John Young's book *Beyond Treatment: Discover How to Build a Cellular Foundation to Achieve Optimal Health*. He takes the reader on a journey through his traditional medical school and residency training.

Equipped with his newfound knowledge of medicine and a bag full of modern miracle medicines he traveled to Swaziland in Southern Africa. His expectation of gaining the appreciation of this poor, rural patient population by bringing them his modern knowledge of medicine to treat common diseases like high blood pressure was quickly dashed. He finds that a man he treated for hypertension with his American-made hypertensive medication not only did not return to his clinic to thank him but later finds that the man went to a witch doctor who provided him with a potion that made him feel better.

With this new perspective on the efficacy of modern medicines for treating illnesses he began to research not only the benefits but also the litany of side effects that are associated with taking the so-called modern miracle drugs. Enter nutrition. It is well documented that at most medical schools, medical students receive no more than a few hours of lectures on the benefits of nutrition and exercise. Dr. Young nicely puts into perspective the need to consider all food groups for a balanced healthy diet. Although fruits and vegetables are certainly healthy, he notes that it should not be at the expense of decreasing protein intake. He documents the relationship between inflammation and autoimmune diseases and cancers and the importance of the essential fatty acids for improving immune function and reducing risk of these chronic illnesses.

Living in sunny Florida, Dr. Young appreciated the fact that most people not only avoided the sun or wore sun protection but were indoors between 10 AM and 3 PM, which are the times when vitamin D production occurs in the skin. Not to his surprise, he found that most of his patients were vitamin D deficient. Getting high doses of vitamin D not only made his patients feel better but reduced risk for upper respiratory tract infections and other chronic illnesses.

After extensive research Dr. Young has designed the Young Health Shake, a special cocktail of non-denatured whey protein, flax seed & cod liver oil and a patented alkalizing mineral blend to provide essential nutrients for the purpose of improving cellular health and immune function. Throughout this book Dr. Young shares fascinating case studies documenting how the Young Health Shake and high-dose vitamin D has helped in treating chronic illnesses including autoimmune diseases, heart disease, asthma and diabetes. I agree with Dr. Young's conclusion "there is no secret formula for restoring health". However there is a formula for maintaining good health as is documented in this book i.e. a well-balanced diet, adequate vitamin D from supplementation and sensible sun exposure and exercise. Those plagued with chronic illnesses can also benefit by following Dr. Young's revolutionary approach to improving cellular and body health.

Introduction

Despite daily bulletins about the dangers of modern medicine and pharmacology, on television and in print, I am feeling more optimistic. The real news is that we have entered a time when hard science is beginning to recognize the relevance of the mind/body connection. Studies are showing that we have the ability to remake our body composition and recognize the power of our mind and heart in that process.

Surprisingly, leaders in physics, cell biology, energy and the new science of epigenetics (meaning *above genetics*, as in "Genes are NOT our destiny"), are producing study after study proving we can change our bodies.

The world of medicine is alive with change. It's a good time to be a physician if you have an energetic, open mind. Thanks to the speed of information technology, doctors and scientists all over the world are sharing discoveries and *Eureka!* moments in real time. Science is moving away from seeing the body simply as a machine, and instead, is recognizing the complexities and capabilities of the human being.

We now understand that we are on an extraordinary voyage. To quote Albert Claude, the 1974 Nobel Laureate in Medicine,

Man is a colony of cells in action. It is the cells, which achieve, through him, what he has the illusion of accomplishing himself. It is the cells, which create and maintain in us...our will to survive, to search and experiment.

It all comes down to basic biochemistry and physiology: how the cells work individually, with the organs, and the body as a whole. Supporting our cells is our first priority—not only for physical health, but for emotional and creative health as well. Every day we have the opportunity to be more of what we were intended to be. Through our ability to question, we can overcome the overwhelming pressure of *Big Pharma* on our political institutions, the communications industry, and our daily interactions with friends, relatives and our doctors. Our cellular structure needs us to be focused and sure about the kind of body we want, the kind of relationships we want, and the kind of message we want to send to the world through our work and creativity.

Just think about that for a minute. Soak it in because once we realize this fact of life, we can consciously act on what we have learned. What a challenge and an opportunity. This book details my journey to that realization and how I am sharing this knowledge with my patients.

.

Section 1

Taking the Alternative Route

1. Living in America:
Habits That Shape Our Overall Health

It's important to start with the truth, and here's a fact we can't deny—Americans are sicker than ever. Though the message of this book is one of hope and actual positive results, we must face the ongoing evidence and overwhelming statistics that show how far down the rabbit hole we have fallen. Then we'll see how I propose to get us back into the sunshine.

In 2005, a report published in *The New England Journal of Medicine* stated that the life expectancy for the average American could decline by as much as five years in the future. According to a team of scientists, supported in part by the National Institute of Aging—a division of the National Institutes of Health of the Department of Health and Human Services—poor lifestyle habits were to blame for the first possible sustained drop in life expectancy in modern times.

And then, just six years later, this prognosis was confirmed: a medical expert at Gottlieb Memorial Hospital, part of the Loyola University Health System, concluded that...

...for the first time in history, the next generation will live two to five years less than their parents.

A similar study released earlier this year stated that Americans are not just in poorer health compared to those around the world, but they're also dying earlier—with the American male ranking at the bottom of the list with a life expectancy of 75.6 years. Even more disheartening: The "mortality gap"—as it was referred to—has been widening for the past three decades.

This report, which was released from the Institute of Medicine and the national Research Council (two non-profit groups that advise the government on health), concludes with the following statement:

"The tragedy is not that the United States is losing a contest with other countries, but that Americans are dying and suffering from illness and injury at rates that are demonstrably unnecessary. Superior health outcomes in other nations show that Americans also can enjoy better health."

So how did we get here? I believe it is due to our on-the-go, quick fix mentality. We have reached this point because we are in the habit of instant gratification. We are a rush society. It just seems easier to pop something in the microwave when we're hungry and to take a medication when we feel sick. So now we are in deep trouble. Short-term fixes are leading to long-term problems.

Frank Jordan, author and international TV, radio and web health talk commentator, agrees with me, adding, "Multiple lifestyle issues have severely impaired our body's ability to maintain and regain proper health." He cites poor diet and nutrition, lack of adequate exercise, sleep deprivation, excess stress, toxic overload, acidity dominance and over-emphasis on prescription drugs as the main culprits.

The good thing is that all of these issues can be addressed between doctor and patient.

2. One Size Does Not Fit All

Imagine that you wake up one morning and don't feel well. The ailment could have any one or more of the following common symptoms: headache, low-grade fever, upset stomach, constipation, aching muscles, sore throat or congestion. Or perhaps you're going about your busy day when all of a sudden one or more of these symptoms strike. Or maybe you live day in and day out with one or more chronic health problems, like back pain, fatigue, insomnia, migraines or difficulty concentrating.

Here's a quiz. What would most likely be your route to wellness?

(a)   Heading to your local pharmacy to scour the shelves for the most appealing yet affordable over-the-counter medicine?

(b)   Calling your doctor with the hope that he or she will write you a prescription?

(c)   Taking an honest inventory of your

lifestyle in order to correct any poor

habits that may be contributing to your

current health issues?

    The truth of the matter is, the majority of Americans will answer either (a) or (b). And that's because we have become accustomed to treating the symptoms instead of searching for the underlying root cause. We have arrived at this point because most people basically look to their doctor to stop their symptoms, but it wasn't always this way.

    Up until the early 1960s, good doctors would research until they discovered an individualized treatment for each sick patient. He or she would then come up with a special formula for the condition or disease they were treating. Doctors would actually create a lot of their own concoctions. But then the pharmaceutical companies started to take over.

The end result has been a one size fits all approach to health and healing. What they did was say, "Here, let's make this a uniform plan for everybody. So instead of Dr. Jones and Dr. Smith having his and her treatment for croup, or a whole group of doctors in town with different treatments for gastritis or strep throat, let's come up with a standard treatment. And we can patent that!" And thus they created Tagamet, Zantac, Nexium, Prilosec, and so on.

These days, it tends to work like this. You meet with your doctor who informs you of the illness or disease you have, and the doctor refers to the Physicians' Drug Reference Book to find out what drug to prescribe you. And that's it.

It's no longer about trying to figure out what's going on in your body. It is simply about treating the symptom.

3. Taking the Alternative Route

I'm not pointing fingers or labeling doctors as good or bad. In fact, I was taught to rely on prescriptions as the path to wellness. Like other medical students, I learned the basics, including biochemistry, physiology and anatomy, and then was 'educated' from drug company representatives who taught about the latest antibiotics and drugs for various chronic conditions, such as hypertension, diabetes and heart disease.

After completing my first two years of medical school, I looked forward to years three and four, when I'd begin working in a hospital doing clinical rounds. I was excited that I could now prescribe drugs. After all, these were to be my 'tools' to address the results of my patients' histories and examinations.

During the first years of my medical career, I discovered that some treatments were definite. For example, the cure for appendicitis was the removal of the appendix. Yet when it came to chronic conditions, the treatment was not nearly as clear.

I went to medical school because I wanted to cure sickness and disease, kind of a novel idea. But I found myself just prescribing any drug I could find that would make my patients' complaints go away.

4. The Witch Doctor

It was four years beyond medical school before I learned my first invaluable lesson about medicine. I was working in Swaziland, a little mountainous kingdom located between Mozambique and the Republic of South Africa. While treating patients in a rural clinic, I was assigned to a man who was complaining about high blood pressure. I took care of this man the only way I knew how—by prescribing him meds made in the United States. Arrogantly, I assumed this man would be very grateful because I had given him an expensive, American-made drug that was highly sought-after in Africa. I told the patient to return for a follow-up appointment in two weeks. He never came back.

As fate would have it, I ran into this patient in town several weeks later. When I asked him why he hadn't come back to see me for the follow up appointment, he looked at me somewhat sheepishly and said, "You never got me better."

"What do you mean I didn't get you better?" I replied. "I gave you the medicine from the United States. It's the best medicine for hypertension! So what did you do?"

The man's answer stunned me. "I went to the witch doctor. He gave me something to drink and now I'm better."

Now I was the sheepish one. My little medical bag of American medicine had just lost out to a witch doctor—the local medicine man—whose only education was what had been passed down to him through generations of traditional African medicine. This was a humbling lesson for an aspiring young doctor, armed with pills, academic degrees and a fragile ego.

5. Daring to Ask a Simple Question

While this particular experience made an impression, I somehow managed to put the witch doctor incident out of my mind. Soon after returning home, I was accepted into an internal medicine residency at the Marshall University School of Medicine where I was required to work at The Veterans Administration Hospital in Huntington, West Virginia. It didn't take me long to notice this hospital had about sixty "revolving door" patients.

On a regular basis, these sixty patients would be hospitalized for a couple of weeks. We'd get them a little better and send them home. In about three or four weeks, they'd come back. We'd treat them again and send them home. Three or four weeks later they'd return again, and the cycle would continue. Somewhere in my education I had been told that the definition of insanity is doing the same thing, over and over, expecting different results. Here was a classic case of that insanity being demonstrated right in front of me.

Something dawned on me while I was treating a very sick—and possibly terminally ill— man. I was doing my residency/specialty training and I had a patient come in who had been to the hospital numerous times for severe lung disease. One day I said to my chief resident as we were treating this man in the intensive care unit: "Bob, have you noticed that Mr. Jones is always in and out of the hospital? What if we tried something really wild? What if we tried to actually *cure* him?"

Bob looked at me and said, "John, are you out of your mind? Do you want to finish your residency?" Of course I said yes, and then he said, "Just shut your mouth and do what everybody else does." So I shut my mouth, did what everybody else was doing and I finished my residency. But inside, it really bugged me that we were pumping people full of drugs and not making any of them better for the long haul.

This experience remained deep within me for the years ahead. I continued my career in the medical field, working in emergency rooms both in America and around the world, while fleeting thoughts of the African man's witch doctor and the lung patient in the ICU returned to me time and time again. I'd keep asking myself if I was really getting people better. After being in practice for a number of years, I just couldn't take it anymore. I knew there had to be a better way to practice medicine.

Your vision will become clear only when you can look into your own heart. Who looks outside, dreams; who looks inside awakens.
Carl Jung

6. What Came First: Problem or Symptom?

To illustrate my point on treating a symptom, consider professional golfer Phil Mickelson. Phil had been diagnosed with psoriatic arthritis—a chronic autoimmune disease, which is a form of arthritis. Prior to the 2010 PGA Championship, Phil announced he had this condition and that he'd been taking weekly shots of the pharmaceutical drug Enbrel, also known as Etanercept, which helps to lower levels of a protein that triggers inflammation. In a press conference, Phil had this to say to a group of golf reporters about his experience with Enbrel: "I feel great. I'm able to work out and don't have any pain. So I've had some good immediate response. And that's why I feel comfortable talking about it, knowing that long-term and short-term, things are fine."

Phil became a spokesperson for this drug because it no doubt made him feel wonderful. Drugs like Enbrel and Humira basically knock out the immune system. And when you knock out the immune system, diseases like psoriatic arthritis and any type of degenerative joint injuries will be managed because the immune system will no longer have the ability to attack against itself. So the pain is gone and the patient feels fantastic.

Here's where we run into a problem. Unfortunately, once you knock out the immune system, your chances of contracting other illnesses, like the flu or pneumonia, greatly increase because your body cannot fight off the infections.

Another disease that may occur from the long-term use of these types of drugs is cancer.

We are seeing huge increases in cancers in those patients who have been taking drugs that destroy the immune system. It's been happening around the eight to ten year mark.

This particular side effect hits really close to home for me. My sister was diagnosed with a type of skin cancer, and she's been on these immune-destroying drugs for years. So what's the current treatment for cancer? Being prescribed radiation and chemotherapy from an oncologist. And the cycle continues.

I can also speak from personal experience as a patient. I was suffering from allergies and was desperate to find a cure. Every winter, from November until April, I'd suffer from a terrible cough. I saw all of the specialists, took all of the steroids, the antibiotics and anything else they prescribed. But the cough persisted.

In desperation, I chose to be pro-active and headed down the non-conventional route. I did some research on my own and elected to have a delayed allergy test, which showed I had a delayed allergy to a pesticide used on produce overseas (a pesticide that is outlawed in the United States). So when would I have eaten produce from overseas? Each year between November and April, we were either getting seasonal produce from overseas or I would take an annual trip to South Africa to visit friends. And when did I have my cough? From November until April, even though it would take about three weeks for the cough to manifest. Bottom line, I had a delayed allergy.

But here's the really interesting part. If you ask most doctors about having a delayed allergy, they will say this condition does not exist. However, if you look up allergies in the Harrison's Textbook of Medicine, it highlights the four different types of allergic reactions: type I is an allergy that develops immediately and up to one hour; type II will develop within hours and up to a few days; type III will reveal itself within a week or weeks; and in type IV, the reaction will become apparent within weeks or even months. And yet, many doctors refuse to believe in a delayed allergy.

Why? The reason is because it cannot be fixed with a standard form of treatment. A delayed allergy is not a type I allergy, and that is the type of allergic reaction where a patient can receive a series of shots that may help the body become immune to the allergen. The treatment for a delayed allergy is nutritional. And if a condition cannot be treated with a prescription drug, then many doctors will deny that the condition and/or the nutritional remedy even exist.

Before we discuss what *can* be done, it's important to look at what stands in the way. The major blocks are money, greed and politics plus something I mentioned earlier—the need for speed.

7. The Pharmaceutical Influence

So why, for the most part, are the majority of medical experts anti-nutrition? The answer is one word: money. Nutrition is not a part of medicine because it is not pharmaceutical. In other words, there is no money to be made in it. The pharmaceutical industry has basically taken over medicine. I'll even go so far as to say that our political system is in bed with the pharmaceutical system, something that is, fortunately, starting to make headlines.

Frank Jordan concurs with me on this. He says, "We, as a nation, have forfeited information and the teaching of critical variables in nutrition, hygiene and disease education to the media, whose content is determined by advertisers and their advertising dollars. And who are the largest providers of advertising dollars? The producers of prescription drugs."

He continues, "I believe the second greatest influence is our government. From schools to federal, the standards of care are archaic and highly prejudiced against the natural versus the synthetic. The emphasis today is on treating symptoms influenced by the pharmaceutical industry and the almighty dollar rather than treating an individual as a unique creature. Natural and nutritional are now the 'alternative' medicines while synthetic substances are the mainstream forms of treatment. The emphasis is on the patentable rather than the effective. And until there is emphasis on determining the cause of a health issue in order to determine a pathway to recovery to or maintenance of good health, I'm sorry to say we are on a dead end street—literally."

My goal, as an aware physician, is to encourage patients and doctors to search for the root cause of the problem. What I ask all of us to do is take a step back from the medications. Let me be very clear—I have no problem with drugs when used properly. For example, I will still prescribe my asthma and emphysema patients an inhaler because I think they can work wonders in an emergency situation.

When it comes to the acute medical problem, I truly believe the American system is the best in the world. If you're having a heart attack, for instance, there is no other place you'd rather be than in the United States. But what we have done in the process is taken a chronic problem and put an acute treatment on them.

Another downside is that health problems are covered up with medications. We are no longer getting people well—it's all symptomatic treatment versus attempting to find the root of the problem. This is the situation we have created in American medicine and this is why we are in trouble.

Section 2

The Solution:

Rebuild your Health at the Cellular Level

8. The Denial Effect

Earlier in this book, Frank Jordan provided a list of factors that are contributing to our nation's deteriorating health: poor diet and nutrition, lack of adequate exercise, sleep deprivation, excess stress, toxic overload, acidity dominance and over-usage of prescriptions drugs. Let's explore each of these items:

Poor Diet and Nutrition: According to a 2010 survey conducted by the United States Department of Agriculture, the average American adult (a 5'9" male weighing 190 pounds; a 5'4" female weighing 164 pounds) consumes 1,996.3 pounds of food each year. While some of the year-end totals are encouraging—415.4 pounds of vegetables and 273.2 pounds of fruit—the majority of the year-end totals are not.

Over the course of one year, the survey states the average American adult consumes: 141.6 pounds of caloric sweeteners; 42 pounds of corn syrup; 29 pounds of French fries; 23 pounds of pizza; 24 pounds of ice cream; 24 pounds of artificial sweeteners; 2.736 pounds of sodium (which is 47% more than recommended), and 53 gallons of soda. In total, Americans eat an average of 2,700 calories each day.

Data collected from the 2005-2007 National Health Interview Survey (NHIS), which is conducted by the Centers for Disease Control and Prevention's National Center for Health Statistics, reported the following: 61.2% of adults were current alcohol drinkers, with nearly one in three reporting five or more drinks in one day during the year; and 20.4% of adults were cigarette smokers, with 16% reporting daily smoking.

As for children eating a poor diet, the problem may begin as early as in the womb. Research published in the March 2013 issue of The Federation of American Societies for Experimental Biology Journal suggests that pregnant women who consume junk food can cause changes in the development of the opioid signaling pathway in the brains of their unborn children. As a result, babies are less sensitive to opioids, chemicals that are released when consuming foods high in fat and sugar. In the long run, these children are born with a higher tolerance to junk food and will need to eat more of it to achieve a feel good response.

Lack of Exercise: According to the National Health Interview Survey, nearly four in ten adults (39.7%) did not take part in any leisure-time physical activity over the course of the year. About one in five adults (21.9%) only engaged in light to moderate leisure-time physical activity.

These factors combined can contribute to a lack of productivity in the workplace, according to a new study published in the October issue of *Population Health Management*. Out of 19,803 employees polled around the country, those with an "unhealthy diet" were 66% more likely to report having experienced a loss in productivity than workers who regularly ate whole grains, fruits and vegetables.

Employees who exercised only occasionally were 50% more likely to report having lower levels of productivity than those who were regular exercisers. And smokers were 28% more likely than non-smokers to report suffering from a drop in productivity.

"Total health-related employee productivity loss accounts for 77 percent of all such loss and costs employers two to three times more than annual healthcare expenses," said lead author Ray Merrill, a Professor in the Department of Health Science, Brigham Young University.

Sleep Deprivation: The National Sleep Foundation states that, according to various studies, every year as many as 58% of American adults report moderate to chronic insomnia and/or sleep related disorders. According to the NHIS survey, almost three in ten adults, or 28%, averaged six hours of sleep or fewer per night.

Lack of adequate amounts of sleep has been linked to very serious health conditions including heart disease, high blood pressure, stroke and diabetes.

Excess Stress: According to the Anxiety and Depression Association of America, anxiety and stress-related disorders affect 40 million adults in the United States, which is 18% of the population. The most common mental illness in the country today, Americans spend more than $42 billion a year treating these disorders. A couple of the conditions that fall under this category include:

Generalized Anxiety Disorder (GAD), which affects 6.8 million adults and is characterized by persistent, excessive, and unrealistic worry about everyday things.

Panic Disorder and Agoraphobia, which affects nearly 6 million Americans and is diagnosed in people who experience spontaneous, seemingly out-of-the-blue panic attacks and are preoccupied with the fear of a recurring attack. Panic attacks, also known as anxiety attacks, occur unexpectedly, sometimes even during sleep.

Anxiety has been implicated in several illnesses such as heart disease, chronic respiratory disorders, and gastrointestinal conditions.

Over-usage of Prescription Drugs (which ties into toxic overload, acidity dominance): According to the latest statistics from the Centers for Disease Control and Prevention, 47.9% of Americans use at least one prescription drug each month; 21.4% use three or more prescription drugs each month; and 10.5% use five or more prescription drugs each month.

About 2.6 billion drugs were prescribed during physician office visits; 255 million drugs were prescribed during hospital outpatient department visits; and 267.7 million drugs were prescribed during hospital emergency department visits.

The Centers for Disease Control and Prevention also released the following information regarding prescription drug use:

Between 1998 and 2008, the percentage of Americans who took at least one prescription drug per month increased from 44% to 48%. The use of two or more drugs increased from 25% to 31%. The use of five or more drugs increased from 6% to 11%.

In 2007 and 2008, two out of every ten children and nine out of ten older Americans reported using at least one prescription drug in the previous month.

The most commonly used types of prescription drugs in the United States by age were:

- Bronchodilators for children aged 0-11
- Central nervous system stimulants for adolescents aged 12-19
- Antidepressants for adults aged 20-59
- Cholesterol lowering drugs for adults aged 60 and over

Among children under age 6, penicillin antibiotics were the most frequently used prescription drugs. Diuretics and β-blockers were also very commonly used drugs in adults and older Americans.

In 2012, *Forbes* magazine sponsored a survey (conducted by Google Consumer Surveys) on a smaller scale (1,073 online responses). However, their results were somewhat similar to those of the Centers for Disease Control and Prevention. According to the *Forbes* online poll:

- 34% of American adults take at least one prescription drug
- 11.5% of American adults take three or more prescription drugs
- 6.5% of American adults take four or more prescription drugs

Lastly, here is the information taken from a press release from the Centers for Disease Control and Prevention dated February 20, 2013. In 2010, nearly 60 percent of the drug overdose deaths (22,134) involved pharmaceutical drugs. Opioid analgesics, such as oxycodone, hydrocodone, and methadone, were involved in about three out of every four pharmaceutical overdose deaths (16,651), confirming the predominant role opioid analgesics play in drug overdose deaths.

The researchers also found that drugs often prescribed for mental health conditions were involved in a significant number of pharmaceutical overdose deaths. Benzodiazepines (antianxiety drugs) were involved in nearly 30 percent (6,497) of these deaths; antidepressants in 18 percent (3,889), and antipsychotic drugs in 6 percent (1,351).

With these statics, we are concerned that 4 people have died of vitamin D overdose in 50 years. We have tried to blackball anyone that does not use pharmaceutical drugs to say how dangerous these non-pharmaceutical drugs are for people. The *statics* show pharmaceutical drugs have killed far more people than the natural products have.

9. Yes, It's Become Chronic

I know this is getting overwhelming, but bear with me for a little longer. We'll get to the good stuff.

So what is the result of all of these negative habits and lifestyle choices? The human body can respond to these harmful factors in different ways, but there are three chronic conditions that have become epidemics in our society: obesity, diabetes and autoimmune diseases.

Obesity

Obesity is determined by using weight and height in order to calculate a number that is referred to as the body mass index (BMI). BMI correlates with a person's amount of body fat. An adult who has a BMI between 25 and 29.9 is considered overweight. An adult who has a BMI of 30 or higher is considered obese.

Keep in mind that BMI is an estimate of body fat and does not directly measure body fat. For example, many athletes have a BMI that categorizes them as overweight, even though they most likely do not have excess body fat.

No matter where you turn, the numbers for obesity continue to rise at alarming rates. A March 2013 statistic released by the World Health Organization claims that, "Obesity has reached epidemic proportions globally, with at least 2.8 million people dying each year as a result of being overweight or obese. Once associated with high-income countries, obesity is now also prevalent in low- and middle-income countries."

If we look closer to home, the numbers are even more staggering. The Centers for Disease Control and Prevention reports a "dramatic increase" in obesity in the United States over the past twenty years. Their latest facts are as follows:

35.7%, or more than one-third of adults in the U.S., are obese. In 2008, medical costs associated with obesity were estimated at $147 billion; the medical costs for people who are obese were $1,429 higher than those of normal weight. "And no state met the nation's Healthy People 2010 goal to lower obesity prevalence to 15%. Rather, in 2010, there were 12 states with an obesity prevalence of 30%."

Complications from obesity include type 2 diabetes, arthritis, coronary heart disease and stroke, hypertension, depression, sleep apnea, gall bladder disease, gynecological problems, sexual health issues, and cancer, including cancer of the uterus, cervix, ovaries, breast, colon, rectum and prostate.

Our children are not exempt! According to data collected from the National Health and Nutrition Examination Survey, approximately 12.5 million, or 17%, of children and adolescents aged two through nineteen are obese, and since 1980, obesity prevalence among children and adolescents has almost tripled.

If Americans continue on this course, by 2030, 13 states could have adult obesity rates above

60%, 39 states could have rates above 50%, and all 50 states could have rates above 44%, according to *F as in Fat: How Obesity Threatens America's Future 2012, a* report released by Trust for America's Health (TFAH) and the Robert Wood Johnson Foundation (RWJF).

This analysis has also predicted that obesity could contribute to more than 6 million cases of type 2 diabetes, 5 million cases of coronary heart disease and stroke, and more than 400,000 cases of cancer in the next two decades. By 2030, medical costs associated with treating preventable obesity-related diseases are estimated to increase by $48 billion to $66 billion per year in the United States, and the loss in economic productivity could be between $390 billion and $580 billion.

In my travels around the world, I am ashamed to say it is only in the United States that I see this terrible epidemic of obesity. It really comes down to this—it is the quality of what we put in our mouths. While people may be exercising more, the epidemic is getting greater and greater.

But it's not only the quality of what someone puts into his or her mouth, but also the quantity that makes a difference. It's been widely reported that portion size has increased significantly over the last two decades. The 2004 documentary *Super Size Me* comes to mind.

Now research is indicating that eating habits, like bigger helpings, may be passed down to our kids. Researchers from Washington State University discovered that mothers who are emotional eaters or have no self-control when it comes to food tend to produce children who have a strong desire to eat—a behavior that may influence a pre-school age child's risk of becoming obese.

When it comes to obesity, your body is producing a lot of insulin to drive the blood sugar into the cells, and you are going to develop something called insulin resistance. Then, after a while, the cells are going to say, "I'm going to need more than just one or two units of insulin to help me get this sugar into the cell. I'm going to need twenty or thirty units of insulin to get these cells in order for the pancreas to make that!" And when the pancreas starts making a lot of insulin, insulin says to the body, "Store fat around the liver, coronary arteries and carotid arteries."

Insulin is also a binder. It binds hormones, like sex hormones and thyroid hormones. It is a pro-aging hormone. It also binds serotonin, dopamine and norepinephrine, which are all connected to depression. So, in other words, insulin in large amounts is not good!

Take a deep breath. We're almost there. I know it's heavy, but we have to understand what's happening in the body in order to know how to approach it. Our bodies are meant to cooperate, but all of these stresses have created a battlefield.

The terms obesity and insulin brings us to the next chronic condition in our society today—diabetes.

Diabetes

Data from the 2011 National Diabetes Fact Sheet reports that 25.8 million children and adults in the United States—which is 8.3% of the population—have diabetes. An alarming 79 million people are suffering from pre-diabetes. Some of the complications from diabetes overlap with the complications from obesity, including heart disease (adults with diabetes have heart disease death rates about two to four times higher than adults without diabetes); stroke (the risk for stroke is two to four times higher among people with diabetes); and high blood pressure (between 2005 and 2008, 67% of adults with diabetes used prescription medications for hypertension). Other common complications include blindness (diabetes is the leading cause of new cases of blindness among adults); kidney disease (diabetes is the leading cause of kidney failure); nervous system disease (between 60% and 70% of diabetic adults have mild to severe forms of nervous system damage); and amputation (more than 60% of non-traumatic lower-limb amputations occur in people with diabetes).

As for the current cost of diabetes, in 2012, the number totaled $245 billion ($176 billion for direct medical costs and $69 billion in reduced productivity).

I treat a large number of type 2 diabetics, and if you refer to the textbooks of physiology and biochemistry, one of the things they talk about in type 2 diabetes is an insulin resistance problem. Again, what that means is the receptors that carry the blood sugar into the cells become resistant, so the body needs more insulin to get the job done. But after a while, the body cannot keep up with the demand, so the next thing you know you're at the doctor's office where he says to you, "Your blood sugar is 300—we're going to put you on some pills or some insulin to drive your blood sugar down."

While this method will work, what happens is that your doctor will continue to add more and more drugs as the years go by. Once again, this brings us back to the whole idea of simply treating the symptom. The approach should be about getting to the root of the problem instead of the doctor saying, "Oh no, your blood sugars are high. Here, take Metformin or take insulin." And in the case of type 2 diabetes, the goal is to reset those insulin receptors.

Recently it came out that researchers expect approximately 30% to 35% of the U.S. population to be diabetic or near-diabetic over the next ten to fifteen years. Changes need to be made, now.

Autoimmune Diseases

Autoimmune disease is a condition where the white blood cells in the immune system overreact to stimuli inside the body, attacking the healthy cells by mistake. With more than eighty different types of conditions that fall under this category, including forms of arthritis (like in the case of Phil Mickelson – psoriatic arthritis), lupus, Graves' disease and Chronic Fatigue Syndrome, the National Institutes of Health (NIH) estimates up to 23.5 million Americans suffer from an autoimmune disease. That's more than those who suffer from cancer (which affects about nine million Americans) and heart disease (which affects about 22 million people in this country). The NIH estimates the annual direct health costs for autoimmune disease to be $100 billion. And according to the Department of Health and Human Services' Office of Women's Health, autoimmune disease and disorders ranked number one in a top ten list of most popular health topics requested by callers to the National Women's Health Information Center.

With so many diseases under the autoimmune umbrella, receiving a proper diagnosis tends to be a time-consuming challenge. Also, the symptoms—like fatigue, muscle aches, low-grade fever—often overlap, adding to the frustration of both the doctor and patient.

We didn't see many of these autoimmune cases twenty-five to thirty years ago—and that's because they were very rare. The new reality is that we are seeing an overwhelming number of these cases today.

So what is the reason behind this growing trend? Clearly, something has changed. But what has changed—and is there anything we can do to reverse it?

The U.S. government's research believes the heightened number of diseases our country is dealing with today is the cause of a toxic environment. There can be multiple factors linked to a toxic environment—chemicals, pollution, viruses, bacteria, gas, even people (emotionally speaking, anyway).

My focus is on a toxic food environment. By one definition, this term refers to a wide range of issues: wide availability of unhealthy foods; the high cost of nutritional food; food advertising aimed at children; and the list goes on. The other definition—or a more specific definition—comes from the Department of Agriculture. If you look at the mineral content of a peach grown in the 1940s and compare it to the mineral content of a peach grown today, there would be a substantial difference.

The difference? You'd need to eat thirty of today's peaches in order to receive the mineral content of a peach grown in the 1940s. It comes down to this—our food has lost its nutritional value, and as a result, our immune systems are not as strong as they were decades ago.

10. Then There's Inflammation

The word inflammation comes from the Latin *inflammo*, meaning, *"I set alight, I ignite"*. According to the website Medical News Today, the definition of inflammation is as follows: *Inflammation is the body's attempt at self-protection; the aim being to remove harmful stimuli,*

*including damaged cells, irritants, or pathogens—
and begin the healing process.*

When we hear the word inflammation, we tend to think of an area that throbs with pain due to some type of accident (like a stubbed toe or a bee sting) or a type of sudden body malfunction (like a toothache, an earache or an allergic reaction on the skin caused by a cream, perfume, laundry detergent, etc.). But what many people fail to realize is that all chronic conditions—whether it be any of the diseases previously mentioned or others, such as asthma, heart disease, or stroke—stem from the same cause: inflammation.

The field of medicine seems to agree that all of the chronic diseases start with an inflammatory process. It is written about in all of the medical journals, and it's been several years since the Australians discovered what they named substance P. This substance seems to initiate the whole inflammatory cascade.

The bottom line is this: all chronic conditions come down to an inflammatory process.

11. The Solution: Rebuild Your Health at the Cellular Level

Now we get to the good part. As I mentioned earlier, my purpose in becoming a doctor was to make sick people better. But as the years progressed, I found that I was routinely prescribing medicine to treat my patients' symptoms. I wasn't actually healing anyone, and I figured the only way I could make that happen was to get to the root of the problem.

Instead of continuing on the same medical path, I decided to study some theories and practices of doctors from the past. I wanted to find out how the greats in medicine treated patients. I immersed myself in the works of Dr. John Myers, a former professor of medicine at John Hopkins University; Otto Warburg, a doctor who won the Nobel Prize in Physiology in 1931; Dr. Robert Cathcart, an orthopedic surgeon who later specialized in allergy, environmental and orthomolecular medicine; and Dr. Johanna Budwig, whose discoveries would eventually have the biggest impact on the way I practice medicine.

I kept reading to find out how these giants in medicine made people better. And what I first learned from reading the literature is this:

As in building a house, it's imperative to lay a basic foundation.

So here we are, laying the foundation of our 'house of health. If you are a conscientious patient—one who looks further than the prescription pad—you are inundated with healers who recommend alternative therapies, especially through the Internet. You are also chastised by those who would tell you that there is no other way but the traditional American medical system. The truth is, there are non-mainstream therapies that have stood the test of time and the clinical review of doctors and scientists. As Dr. Dan C. Roehm, M.D. FACP (Oncologist and Cardiologist) says about his research into the Budwig Protocol that is the foundation of my Young Health Shake:

"I only wish that all my patients had a PhD in Biochemistry and Quantum Physics to enable them to see how, with such consummate skill, this diet was put together. It is a wonder."

In 1931, Dr. Otto Warburg won the Nobel Prize in Medicine for demonstrating that, unlike normal cells, which receive their energy from oxygen gas, the energy that maintains cancer cells is derived principally from the fermentation of glucose. In his words:

"Cancer, above all other diseases, has countless secondary causes. But, even for cancer, there is only one primary cause. Summarized in a few words, the prime cause of cancer is the replacement of the respiration of oxygen in normal body cells by a fermentation of sugar (glucose)...All cancer cells without exception must ferment, and no normal growing cell ought to exist that ferments in the body."

It is shocking to realize that the world-famous organization that awards the Nobel prizes recognized the value of this research into the healing of cancer, and yet we continued on the course of radiation, chemotherapy and deadly drugs. As always, I value the contributions of traditional medicine. However, to set aside such a significant discovery is not smart medicine.

The renowned German scientist, Dr. Johanna Budwig (pharmacist, researcher, and chemist with a doctorate in Physics), was familiar with the work of Dr. Warburg and had been conducting many studies that confirmed his findings, which were not limited to cancer. Just imagine—she warned us about the dangers of hydrogenated oils in the 1930s! Though she documented multiple cases of cancer being reversed through her "Budwig Cocktail", she believed that addressing the level of cellular healing affected every area of human health. She has been quoted as saying: "The body, soul, mind and spirit all have their functions and roles to play. But the harm done by eating the wrong kind of food fats has repercussions in all realms of life, including healthy mental and spiritual functioning." Though Dr. Budwig was denied her stature in the traditional medical field—due, some say, to her refusal to turn her procedure into an expensive protocol—her influence has not waned. More and more evidence points to her being ahead of her time.

In 1998, the Nobel Prize in Physiology and Medicine was awarded jointly to Robert F. Furchgott, Louis J. Ignarro and Ferid Murad, "…for their discoveries concerning nitric oxide as a signalling molecule in the cardiovascular system." Other research followed which determined the importance of nitric oxide as a signal molecule that is of key importance to the cardiovascular system and many other systems—a signal molecule in the nervous system, a weapon against infections, a regulator of blood pressure and a gatekeeper of blood flow to different organs. As experts since Dr. Budwig have confirmed, it is the protein in the shake (in this case the Young Health Shake developed by me and used in my protocol) that helps the body make nitric oxide. The muscles use this to make more nitric oxide, creating a cascade of healing in the nervous system and the other systems mentioned above.

In 1999, Günter Blobel received the Nobel Prize in Medicine, "…for the discovery that proteins have intrinsic signals that govern their transport and localization in the cell." His findings show the importance of proteins and how the body uses them. This led to my insistence on a strong amino acid profile in my shake. Everything in my protocol is an essential ingredient, backed by solid, Nobel Prize-winning science.

The next step was to figure out exactly what my foundation would consist of. I did a lot of reading and also talked to a number of these doctors. I decided that the foundation for my practice in medicine was going to be basic biochemistry and physiology— meaning how the body works—by getting down to the level of the molecules and the biochemistry of the cells and how they interact.

Then I added the final piece to my new medical foundation. I based my purpose on the 1931, the 1998 and the 1999 Nobel Prizes in Medicine. I affirmed that I was now going to practice medicine from a scientific standpoint, not from a drug company standpoint.

As mentioned earlier, all health issues begin with an inflammatory process. The goal is to stop and then reverse that process. It comes down to this—treat the cell, restore the body. This statement holds true for every illness and disease. I can't think of a single condition where the cells are not involved. Even an injury, like an automobile accident, comes down to breakage of tissues and the breakage of cells. I want to give my patients the best cell membranes and the best immune system possible. In order to do that, I need to help them remake those cell membranes.

During my research, I continually came across the 1931 Nobel Prize in Medicine, which specifically talked about inflammation. More than seventy years ago, a German biochemist named Dr. Johanna Budwig offered her findings for what she believed was the root cause of cancer—when the oxygenation in a cell drops below 35 percent.

What she realized was that in order to keep the oxygen within the cell above 35 percent, you have to remake that cell membrane into a CIS-membrane. This means it has a positive charge on the outside and a negative charge on the inside. It acts like a magnet by pulling oxygen off the red blood cells, which increases the oxygenation.

Dr. Budwig's findings led to the creation of The Budwig Cocktail, which is a simple mixture of an omega-3 essential fatty acid with a protein. But here's the trick: in order for the body to absorb the omega-3 oil it must be emulsified in the protein! Think about it like this, when you eat fish and you cut the fish open, there isn't oil spraying everywhere, because the oil is in the meat, in the protein.

However, when it comes to remaking the cell membranes, all omega-3 oils are not created equal. I learned from the German scientists that flaxseed oil has the most double bonds per molecule, and the cell membranes in our bodies are double-bonded. Also, Americans are up to 80 percent *good fat deficient*. In general, good fats from sources like flax and fish oil modulate inflammation. When we consume oil on its own, our body sees it as a fat, secretes bile, and it breaks down, largely unused.

However, the heart of Dr. Budwig's discovery was that you can cloak that good fat in protein and fool the body to optimize good fat levels. Working with this knowledge, I created a special cocktail using Dr. Budwig's protein and oil formula as the model for The Young Health Shake. Whether they had chronic sore throat, diabetes or cancer, I had all of my patients start with this foundation.

The result? Lo and behold, they started to get better. They would come back to my office in just a couple of weeks and say, "John, I feel really good! My blood sugar is going down, my blood pressure went down, my fatigue is getting better and I need less medication." In other words, The Young Health Shake was bringing down their inflammatory response by remaking the cell membrane. For average Americans, simply taking a vitamin or drug is not going to remake a cell membrane. A great number of my patients are amazed at their poor health, even though they believe they are eating a well-balanced diet. I have a patient who said to me, "Doc, I exercise like crazy and I eat great! In the morning, I have organic oatmeal. For lunch, I have organic salad with fruit. For dinner, I have vegetables and maybe two ounces of range-free chicken." I've heard similar comments many times.

Here's the problem. In this country, we think a healthy diet means eating a lot of fruits and vegetables. We have forgotten the protein. Our immune system is made up of all proteins, our bones are 40 percent protein, and every cell membrane in our body is 60 percent protein. If it were up to me, I would have had Skittles take care of everything. But we need protein.

According to the physiology textbook guidelines, each day your body requires 1 gram of protein for every 2.2 pounds of your body weight, though I never give a patient more than 100 grams of protein in a day.

Here's another helpful guide when figuring out your daily diet: an egg equals roughly 8 grams of protein, and 8 ounces of fish, chicken, beef, or pork, etc. equals approximately 30 grams of protein.

When it comes to diet, vegetables are fantastic. Vegetables have fiber and minerals, which are both very important. And vegetables break down to the carbohydrates sugar. I love carbohydrates—we need carbohydrates. It's just that we have gone too heavy with the carbohydrates and we have forgotten the protein.

As natural as this approach may be, my approach is not a strictly nutritional one. It's just basic biochemistry and physiology. It includes the minerals, the vitamins, the proteins, and the essential fatty acids that make the immune system stronger. These are the building blocks that make up our basic sciences. And it's these basic sciences that have been neglected in medicine today.

It's been nearly ten years since I incorporated this basic foundation, the Young Health Shake, into my practice. It has changed *everything*. Earlier in my career when I worked in the emergency room, I just hated seeing people with these chronic illnesses. But now, I love it—because I can actually do something with these patients! I can usually get them better.

12. Cellular Health: It's Cocktail Time

You have just read about the importance of remaking the cell membranes with my doctor-developed protocol—a concept I call "laying a foundation." I'm going to share with you the components of the Young Health Shake, why it works, and how this cocktail has benefited patients with a wide range of conditions.

What is the Young Health Shake?

When it comes to my patients, it doesn't matter whether they have athlete's foot, gray hair or cancer, I first lay the foundation. As I said earlier, and it bears repeating, it's like building a house— you start out with a foundation, and then you go from there. My job is to give my patients the best immune system and the best cellular health possible. Doctors and researchers have known for decades that a healthy cell structure means a healthier life.

In order to do this, I suggest to all of my patients that they start with "the cocktail," otherwise known as the Young Health Shake. This shake has been designed to remodel and strengthen cell membranes. Based on protocols originally recognized by the Nobel Prize for Medicine in 1931, which I noted earlier, combined with the most thorough medical and physiological research, the cocktail utilizes omega-3 oils emulsified in the highest quality protein to dramatically improve the cells in the body. When your cellular foundation is healthier, your entire body is healthier.

The shake is specifically engineered to deliver inflammatory benefits, which is why it contains high amounts of omega-3-6-9 oils. When the oil is emulsified in a serving that contains twenty-five to thirty grams of a low-heat protein (our protein is never exposed to temperatures over 130 degrees), the cell membranes become more permeable to oxygen.

Now let me explain the importance of low-heat protein. The majority of the whey proteins sold on the market today—at the large vitamin chains or the local health food stores—are heated to about 200 degrees. At that high temperature, all of the health benefits in whey go up in smoke. But a lab figured out to how to heat protein at just 130 degrees, and we have access to this specialized process.

*What can you expect from drinking this
special cocktail? A reduction of the inflammatory
process, which results in healthier, more efficient
cells.*

The Young Health Shake is comprised of
three main ingredients:

Young Health Whey Protein: This protein is
the finest non-denatured (cold processed) native
whey protein concentrate available. It is the optimal
nutritional supplement to assist in antioxidant
production, healthy immune system function,
cellular repair, and it provides all of the amino acids
the body is comprised of. It also aids in muscle
growth and weight management. The polypeptides
in Young Health's whey are critical for proper
organ function, as well as proper food fueling. It is
rich in immunoglobulins and lactoferrin and free of
artificial flavors and sweeteners. The milk used to
create this protein is derived from cows that are
grass fed year round on natural pastures that are
pesticide and chemical free.

For those who may have milk allergies or sensitivities we also produce an Egg White protein that is a sufficient substitute for the preferred whey.

Young Health Flax Seed and Fish Oil Blend:
This oil is a blend of the two most important dietary oils—flaxseed oil and cod liver oil. Flaxseed oil contains the omega fatty acids that the body requires for optimal health, such as the essential fatty acid alpha-Linolenic acid (ALA), which the body converts into Eicosapentaenoic acid (EPA) and Docosahexaenoic acid (DHA), the omega-3 fatty acids found in fish oil. I'm remaking a cell membrane. I need as many double bonds as possible. Flax Oil has the most double bonds per molecule.

Cod liver oil is a great source of vitamins A and D and the omega fatty acids EPA and DHA, which can help nourish the body when attacked by conditions like cardiovascular disease, cancer, diabetes, arthritis, and neurological illnesses like Alzheimer's and autism.

Young Health Balance Drops: Made from calcium chloride, magnesium sulfate, sodium, sulfated castor oil and ultra pure water, these drops are designed to maximize mineral absorption, as well as raise the pH levels in the body, which makes it easier for the blood to give oxygen to a cell. The drops help the body maintain the acid/base (AB) balance in blood and other tissues and produce more bicarbonate (a buffer in the body which prevents blood from becoming too acidic). If acid levels rise and the body cannot produce enough bicarbonate, the body will take alkaline minerals from the bones, leading to osteoporosis.

Recommended Flavoring Techniques:

Fruit of the Spirit - This is a highly concentrated whole fruit puree that is rich in antioxidants and alkalizing minerals. One ounce in the shake adds great flavoring and delivers the nutritional equivalent of five servings of fruits and vegetables.

Fresh or Frozen Berries - A handful of blueberries, strawberries or raspberries will add flavoring and healthy anti-oxidants.

Unsweetened Vanilla or Chocolate Almond Milk
- Adds a nice consistency to the shake. Almond milk is derived from almonds. Almonds are among the healthiest nuts in the world.

For additional flavoring & recipe ideas visit **www.YoungHealth.com**.

13. The Post-Cocktail Effects

Once this foundation is established, around 80 percent of my patients will tell me their problems have greatly diminished. The remaining 20 percent will report an overall improvement, but they still have some remaining issues to deal with and want to feel even better. This is why a lab report is so important. For someone who is not where he or she wants to be in terms of health, I will break him or her down bio-chemically in order to determine what else their body requires.

In these types of cases, I look into adding certain vitamins and minerals to their daily regime. One of the first deficiencies I check for is vitamin D. I have studied and adopted the research of Professor Michael F. Holick, a physician-scientist who is considered a worldwide expert on vitamin D supplementation. As the Director of the General Clinical Research Unit at Boston University, Professor Holick has authored more than 400 publications about the biochemistry, physiology, metabolism and photobiology of vitamin D. He has concluded that vitamin D deficiency is one of the most unrecognized medical conditions. Not only can it leave millions of people at risk for osteoporosis and bone fractures, but it can be a factor in numerous serious and sometimes fatal diseases, such as heart disease, infectious diseases, autoimmune diseases, and various cancers. He even told me recently that vitamin D can cause a cancerous cell to revert back to a normal cell.

Another area I will examine is determining how the body makes energy—a function that is called the Krebs Cycle. Named after a German-born British biochemist, the Krebs Cycle is defined simply by the Random House Kernerman Webster's College Dictionary as the metabolic sequence of enzyme-driven reactions by which carbohydrates, proteins and fatty acids produce carbon dioxide, water and ATP (which stands for Adenosine triphosphate, a coenzyme used as an energy carrier in the cells of all known organisms).

In more basic terms, the Krebs Cycle is where you take in food and it runs through a multiple step process to produce energy. If this cycle does not run effectively, the body will only produce smaller amounts of energy. In other words, this person is not processing their food well, and as a result, their body may store all of that excess food as fat.

I will also check a patient's fasting insulin levels in order to find out how much insulin their body is producing. If they are producing more than four units of insulin, their body will burn muscle and store fat. Along these lines, I'll also look into any possible toxicity issues, as well as how the body absorbs protein and amino acids, along with other possible deficiencies. Once I have broken down my patient bio-chemically and gathered all of this information, I will then add the vitamins, minerals and/or prescriptions necessary.

My goal is to make their regime as simple and affordable as possible. Many of my patients will bring a shopping bag filled with supplements during their office visit, and I will tell them that I can make a case for every product in the health food store. There's only one problem: you will not have enough time in the day to take everything—and you will probably not have enough money to buy everything. Once again, I focus on the basic building blocks derived from the giants in medicine and then, if necessary, make adjustments to suit my patients' individual needs.

For a better understanding of how this protocol works, let's look at 5 types of patients with chronic conditions.

Patient Type #1: Arthritis

I had a female patient in my office who was suffering from polymyalgia rheumatica. Think of it as having arthritis in every single joint in your body. She would tell me that even opening her mouth would be painful and that something as simple as rolling over in bed would cause her to cry out in pain. There wasn't one part of her body that didn't hurt.

During our conversation, she told me about her diet—and I realized that she was eating so many things that were pro-inflammatory. With any type of arthritis, the goal is to stop the inflammatory cascade. So I told her that I wanted to start her out on the Young Health Shake. I advised her to take this cocktail twice a day, each serving containing 30 grams of the low-heat whey protein mixed with one tablespoon of flaxseed oil. I explained that taking an omega-3 supplement on its own would not be beneficial because the body cannot fully absorb the oil unless it is emulsified in a protein.

Two weeks later she returned to my office for a follow-up visit. She shared with me some other health issue she wanted to focus on and I said, "Wait a minute—the last time you told me your biggest problem was polymyalgia rheumatica. You had explained in great detail about the pain you dealt with every single day."

And she said, "Oh, John, the pain has disappeared, just like you said it would!" Let's work on another one of my physical complaints.

Patient Type #2: Asthma

I've had a number of patients who suffered from asthma. As with other chronic diseases, emphysema and COPD (chronic obstructive pulmonary disease), it all comes down to an inflammatory state. Perhaps there's inflammation in the bronchial tubes or the air sacs in the lungs.

Once again, I offered them the Young Health Shake—loading them with the protein and oil combination—along with adding vitamin C to their regime because it's a membrane stabilizer. In other words, it acts like a steroid without being a steroid.

As we know, the drug companies rely on inhalers, a.k.a. the little puffers. While they can work for a time, they tend not to be as effective over time. Again, these inhalers only treat the symptom and they do absolutely nothing to solve the problem.

Within a few weeks' time, most of my asthma sufferers have reported not only felling better, but they have decreased their usage of inhalers. I'm not saying their lungs have completely healed, but they are definitely better.

Patient Type #3: Heart Disease

When it comes to heart disease, it begins with an inflammatory aspect within the coronary arteries, which then leads to plaque buildup. This type of condition brings me to the work of Dr. William Castelli, who had become the third director of the famous Framingham Heart Study in 1979 and who is also a professor of preventative medicine at Harvard Medical School. His studies revealed that people with the lowest cholesterol had the most heart attacks, and the people with vitamin C levels of 3 gm to 5 gm had the fewest heart attacks. It's a vitamin C problem—that's because vitamin C can reduce inflammation, which aids in repairing coronary arteries.

One of my patients, a 79-year-old lady, complained of fatigue and lack of energy. She was diagnosed with atrial fibrillation (an irregular heart beat, also known as A-fib), congestive heart failure, an enlarged heart and high blood pressure. The first thing I did was establish a foundation, which in this case, included the Young Health Shake and iodine.

Iodine is a regulator—it can regulate the thyroid, adrenals, pancreas, ovaries, breast tissue, and it also regulates the heart's electrical system. Some anti-arrhythmic drugs contain large amounts of iodine.

Ten weeks later, we ordered a chest x-ray for her—and the cardiologist stated that the enlarged heart was now a healthy, normal size. He had never seen anything like it before in his entire life!

Fast-forward another eight months and we sent the now 80-year-old lady back to her cardiologist for another reevaluation. The atrial fibrillation, the high blood pressure, it all went away. And this doctor stated that this lady's heart is working like that of a 30-year-old. Needless to say, she was taken off all of her heart medications.

This case can refer back to the 1998 Nobel Prize in Medicine, which states that the muscles surrounding an artery create a gas called nitrous oxide. When the muscles make nitrous oxide, it causes the blood vessels to expand. When the blood vessels expand, the blood pressure drops. In order to make nitrous oxide, you need 1 gm of protein for every 2.2 pounds of body weight. This is another study that backs up the theory that in order to repair anything, you need protein.

Patient Type #4: Diabetes

I treat a tremendous amount of type 2 diabetes patients. Again, referring back to the textbooks of physiology and biochemistry, one of the main factors they discuss about this condition is the insulin resistance problem. In other words, the receptors that carry the blood sugar into the cells become very resistant. As a result, the body needs more insulin in order to get sufficient blood sugar into the cells.

After a while, the body cannot keep up. In most cases, these people will walk out of their doctor's office with a prescription for diabetic pills or insulin to drive the blood sugar down. While the drugs and the insulin will work, these types of treatments are not getting to the root of the problem. It's just another way to treat the symptom. The actual problem is covered up, and as the patient gets older, the doctors will give these patients more and more medications.

The only way to treat an insulin resistance problem is to reset the insulin receptors. I've found that the insulin receptors can be reset using the Young Health Shake protocol.

An insurance company representative recently contacted me and asked, "How do you get so many of your diabetic and hypertension patients off their meds, while the other doctors don't?" Once again, it all comes back to protein.

When I talk about my diabetes patients, I immediately think of a man who came into my office a few years ago. He's a body builder and weight lifter who was in phenomenal shape—but he was suffering from diabetes and even with the meds he was prescribed, his blood sugars were regularly between 250 and 350, which was terrible.

He said to me, "But John, I don't need to take your protein. I'm already drinking protein shakes every day. In fact, I'm consuming 300 grams of protein every day!"

So I responded, "You're coming to see me and your numbers are not good. It's not just about drinking any protein shake, but a whey protein shake where the whey was cooked at a low heat." I asked him to be open-minded and try my regimen for six weeks.

Thankfully, he did. Six weeks later, he returned to my office and tests revealed his blood sugars went way down. Like many other patients of mine, he turned to me and said, "Okay, John—now I understand."

Several years ago, a survey conducted in Tampa Bay revealed some interesting results: 47%

of the people polled said they'd seek the help of an alternative doctor, if given the choice. Times are changing. People are changing. And that's a good thing.

Overall, I look at medicine like this—you know what you're going to get from the general medical community. I'm just one of those doctors who dares to say, "Maybe we can do better."

14. Dr. Young's Six Health Guidelines

Guideline #1: If you have had every medical test known to mankind and seen every specialist and you are *still* not feeling well, take a delayed allergy test. Keep in mind most allergists deny that a delayed allergy test even exists. Therefore, you may need to visit with an alternative physician.

Guideline #2: The reason you go to a doctor is to get better. If you are not getting better, you may need to change physicians. If you brought your car to the same mechanic three times and the car continued to break down, would you keep bringing your car back to this person? Certainly we can agree that your body is more important than your car. Treat your body the way it deserves to be treated.

Guideline #3: Just because your doctor is unsure of your symptoms does not mean they do not exist. It simply means he or she has not researched your condition enough. Do some research yourself. Take control by becoming your own health advocate.

Guideline #4: If your doctor cannot figure out your problem, it does not mean you are suffering from depression. While depression is a very real problem and the effects from depression can be physical, not everyone is suffering from it. Listen to your body. No one knows it better than you.

Guideline #5: If your doctor has not heard of a new treatment or way of treating you, tell him or her to check it out. Your doctor works for you. The majority of doctors will say something like, "I've already spoken to the drug rep and there are no answers." And if your doctor is unwilling to dig deeper, it's probably time to find yourself a new physician.

Guideline #6: Just because the big drug companies do not have a pharmaceutical to treat the condition does not mean you cannot be treated. There are non-pharmaceutical prescriptions and alternative remedies available such as change in diet, supplements, acupuncture, osteopathy, homeopathy, chiropractic treatment, stress management—and the list goes on.

15. A Word On Vitamin D

My goal, as I have said earlier, is to give my patients the best cell membrane and immune system they can have. Besides giving my patients protein to rebuild the immune system, we need one very important vitamin and that's vitamin D. Actually, it's not a vitamin but a hormone. Known as the "sunshine vitamin", you would think that, living in Florida, most of my patients would have plenty of vitamin D. That's not the case. Most people work indoors and they do not go out between 10 a.m. and 2 p.m., which is the best time to create Vitamin D. Also, if you use sun block or long sleeves to protect your skin from the sun, you won't create much vitamin D. I had a patient with a great tan who biked the local bicycle trail three to four times a week so I was positive she had a good vitamin D level. Wrong; it was below the level recommended by the International Organization of Medicine.

The recommended level is 60 units, the level at which the body has the most cancer protection. So I had to supplement her with vitamin D. Levels of vitamin D are either reported as 0 to 29, which is very low, or 30 to 100, which is acceptable. Anything over 100 is considered toxic. That is until I heard a lecture by Professor Michael F. Holick, Ph.D., MD, of Boston University School of Medicine, who said there is no such thing as toxic levels of vitamin D. However, vitamin D can raise calcium levels so you need to watch this. I started to increase my patients' vitamin D levels. As I did, I noticed some interesting things happening.

I had a lady who I put on vitamin D because her level was well below 30. I put her on 20,000 units a day for three months. 20,000 units a day for a month will raise levels by 20 points, and later I decreased her to 10,000 units a day to maintain her level.

The average person uses 5,000 to 10,000 units a day just to live on planet Earth. If they are under a lot stress, they may need 15,000 units a day. Well, my patient misunderstood me and after three months she continued to take 20,000 units of vitamin D a day, month after month. She came in for a checkup and her level was 150! I asked how she felt and she said, "I feel smarter and my hand and eye coordination is better. Also, by the way, I'm never sick." Her calcium levels were fine. I just kept her at that level and she is doing well.

I had another patient with a high level of vitamin D who went to see her pulmonologist. When he saw the level, he stopped her vitamin D immediately, and a few weeks later she ended up in the hospital with pneumonia. She was mad. She fired her pulmonologist and went back on her vitamin D. She has not been sick since.

A little trick I learned: if I feel I'm coming down with a cold, I'll take 40,000 units of vitamin D at bedtime. The next morning, I usually feel like a new person.

An October 2013 study released by Loyola University in Chicago revealed that when 50,000 units of vitamin D *a week* were taken, there was a dramatic reduction in Diabetic Neuropathy after 6 months. I, unfortunately, read the article incorrectly, believing the dose was 50,000 units *a day* so that was what I did. I was checking the calcium levels every month and lo and behold the patient's levels where at 200 points and the neuropathies whether caused by Diabetes or chemotherapy, were either gone or remarkably better after six to eight weeks!

Then I started to look at some autoimmune systems like Rheumatoid Arthritis (RA) and felt that if I could make the immune system more alert, these diseases might respond better to treatment. I had a 26 year old with sever RA. She was on prescription drugs but not doing well when she came to me for help. I started her on the Young Shake to help reduce inflammation, and then put her on a high dose of vitamin D. With her vitamin D levels over 200 within six weeks, she was off all her prescriptions, and feeling great. The Rheumatoid nodules on her bones also started to go away.

There are many stories like this from my practice but what I want to emphasize is that to have a working immune system, one needs vitamin D in larger doses than most doctors are giving.

Now what is even more amazing is that when you combine a low heat protein with flax oil you turn each cell membrane into what we call a CIS configuration: A+ charge on the outside and a negative charge on the inside. Like a battery (what I call the Young Shake), when sunlight hits those positive charges they vibrate and turn mechanical energy into chemical energy called Vitamin D!

Dr. Budwig discussed that many people with a good cell membrane (CIS) would not burn in the sun because, if the cells can vibrate, they react like popcorn. Leave it on the stove and popcorn burns; move it over the kitchen stove top and it does not! Most Americans have Trans Cell Membranes: A+ charge on the inside and a negative charge on the outside cell membrane so they can't vibrate. As a result, the patient's skin burns and they don't make vitamin D. A person with a CIS membrane can make anywhere from 30,000 to 50,000 units of vitamin D per hour if out in direct sunlight.

If you do decide to take high doses of vitamin D, consult with your doctor. But you will be surprised with the results.

Section 3

Client Testimonials

17. Conversation with Dr. Young and Dr. Karin Hotchkiss, pediatric ENT specialist

Karin:

Our story starts seven years ago on a Thursday morning. I was in the operating room when my husband, John, called. He knew it was my operating time, so I knew he wouldn't call unless it was something really urgent. I could tell by his voice something was very wrong. He told me that our daughter, Joy, who was two years old at the time, couldn't walk.

He said she was crying, in a tremendous amount of pain and could not get out of bed. John was carrying her around the house and she wouldn't let him put her down. He was terrified.

Up until that morning, Joy had been a perfectly normal two-year-old. She was running and playing, doing all of the normal things kids her age

can do and meeting all of her developmental
milestones.

We found she had a lot of swelling in one of
her knees, and the initial diagnosis was a septic
joint. We thought she might have a rare infection,
maybe from a cold, and that something had settled
in the joint. Joy spent three weeks on a pick line
with IV antibiotics, and then continued taking
multiple tests and having multiple treatments. We
met with an infectious disease doctor who said, "I
don't think this is infectious—let's look for some
inflammatory markers."

After three months of doctors' visits, Joy
was finally diagnosed with a severe case of juvenile
arthritis. Pediatric rheumatologists are actually a
rare sub-specialty, and at the time there were only
three providers in the state. The entire situation was
frustrating, especially for a mother who is in
medicine where I specialize in pediatric sub-
specialties. This was just off my radar.

For the next seven years, we were in and out
of medical institutions seeking answers from
various specialists. We were there not only to
address her arthritis, but all of the other issues that

went with it: constipation, poor weight gain, physical therapy issues, weak motor tone, like difficulty holding a pencil (a condition which led us to occupational therapy) and emotional issues (which led us to counseling).

After being on medications like Enbrel® (a prescription that treats autoimmune diseases) for six to seven years, John and I realized she was burning out of the biologics. This means that medications can stop working after they've been taken for four to five years. Now we were at the point where everything stopped working. Joy was on the last class of medication, which was Remicade® (another drug that treats various autoimmune diseases) and that wasn't working either. We were beside ourselves.

Every other week, we went for eight-hour infusions at a university that was about two hours away. In between sessions, we were bandaging her pain symptoms—because Joy was in acute pain— with high dose Prednisone (a corticosteroid), which was making her horribly irritable and fussy. She had the classic "moon face" that we talk about when people take high dose steroids.

We asked Joy twice a day, morning and night, to label her pain, and we scaled it on one to ten. For the most part, she was at a ten. Actually, she would say, "Mom, my pain is a 27 out of 10!" and she had been at this pain level for nearly four weeks.

She was screaming, crying and could not get comfortable, even with prescription pain medication. She was absolutely miserable and would say things like, "Why me? This isn't fair." Imagine a parent trying to answer these questions. The pain was also giving her night terrors, and if she was up, we were up.

Along the way, we learned that most types of juvenile arthritis will burn out as the children get older and hit puberty. But Joy had the type that wouldn't burn out—her condition was described as lifelong. Knowing this, and then hearing about how her medications had already exhausted themselves, we felt as if there wasn't a lot of hope. It was a very dark time for our family. We were desperate and at the end of our line, especially because everything that I had read or had been taught as a doctor wasn't working.

The side-effect profile for her diagnosis included cancer. Would she get cancer as a teenager? It was very scary and very real.

My husband and I had then talked about some alternative medication pathways, like acupuncture, and even a method known as iridology—reading past, current and future health issues in the iris of the eye. This practitioner was in North Carolina, and I knew I was ready to try anything

Before that happened, John came home and told me to cancel everything for the following day because he had made an appointment with this man named Dr. Young. It's very rare that I ever cancel my clinics, but I was a desperate mom and this was a day that took precedence.

Before walking through the door of Dr. Young's clinic, my husband and I made a deal—I was going to play the quiet mom and not say a word and he was going to do all of the talking. We felt that would be the best method because I didn't want to bring any bias to the table.

I went into the clinic that day with healthy skepticism—but I also knew we had nothing else going for us. If this was a glimmer of hope, I was going to try it. We knew it was a long shot, but at least we had a shot—and that was more than we had before walking in.

Dr. Young:

As I was listening to Joy's history during her first examination, I thought to myself, "inflammatory aspect." I asked Karin and John "What does Joy eat?"

Karin:

I remember this moment very vividly because I thought, "Oh great, what does she eat?" We knew she didn't have a good diet, and I was going to have to acknowledge that. Joy was suffering from chronic constipation, plus she is naturally thin, so weight was always an issue for her. As parents, we were just happy if she'd eat anything and with all the other issues, we'd feed her whatever she was willing to eat.

Dr. Young:

I listened to this and I thought, "They're feeding this kid everything that is pro-inflammatory!" Joy had already been given a diagnosis of pediatric polyarticular arthritis, which is very rare. I had never treated this condition before, but inflammation is inflammation. Everything she was eating—like macaroni and cheese, which turns to sugar—was just feeding the flame.

So I went back to basics—laying a foundation. I described cell membranes and how they're double-bonded with positive charges on the outside and negative charges on the inside. I also explained that I wanted to test Joy's vitamin D levels.

And, then, Karin asked me a question that I wouldn't expect the average patient to ask. And then another question, and that's when I asked what she did for a living. When she told me she was in the medical profession, I thought, "Oh brother! Another doctor!"

And then I asked, "What do you think of what I've said so far?" And to my surprise, she said, "I think you're right!"

Karin:

I was so enthralled after the first hour that I couldn't stop asking questions! I was intrigued by what Dr. Young had to say because it was everything we had learned from first and second year of medical school. All that was eventually pushed aside because the drugs took over. Interestingly enough, the last appointment we had with Joy's rheumatologist, my husband had asked if diet played any role in this disease—and the doctor told us absolutely not.

We had heard it said that it all comes down to what you put into your body, but when we asked the leading authority who had been our sole provider—and almost rescuer—for the last six years, he told us that diet played no role in Joy's condition. Diet was something we put out of our minds until we met Dr. Young.

After the initial appointment with Dr. Young, we took a closer look at Joy's diet and realized how everything she was eating turned to sugar. Dr. Young even had a diagram in his office showing how much sugar is in the average product. It's just amazing how much sugar is in our food. I was shocked to see there's almost a cup of sugar in steel cut oats. So we really took an inventory on how much sugar Joy was putting in her body. It was almost poison for her.

Dr. Young:

It was interesting, once Karin told me she was a physician, I remember feeling that little swallow in my throat. But then I thought to myself, "Wait. Everything I am doing is in the textbooks of medicine, so there is nothing she could argue with!"

After I finished her physical, I made Joy a shake—this is something I do for all my patients. When I'm dealing with kids, I'm always worried about one thing—are they going to like it? As we all know, you can have the greatest treatment, but if you can't get it in the patient, it's pointless.

I was relieved to find Joy liked it! At this point, I remember thinking, "So far, so good."

Karin:

Once we left Dr. Young's office, we were so excited—all hands on deck! We were in a desperate place. Being in the healthcare business, I felt like I had pulled every string I could pull and I had researched everything I thought I could research. We had come to where we didn't have a lot of hope left, so it was so uplifting as we walked out of the office that day feeling like there was hope after all. We were committed.

When I thought about it, everything Dr. Young had said made sense. Since Joy's diet was extremely poor, we knew that was something we could improve. I remembered Dr. Young had said, "Just get the good stuff in and later we'll worry about weaning off the other things." But as far as we were concerned, we were ready to go cold turkey.

Even better, Joy was on board! I had to hand it to our daughter, at only nine years of age she really stepped up to the plate and became educated on what she could and could not eat.

During the first week, we were very rigid and by-the-book when it came to making the shake—just the protein, the drops and the oil. The nice thing about this product is that it contains an adequate amount of protein but it's low in sugar, unlike some of the big brand, pre-made shakes. But Dr. Young had said, "If you have to sweeten it, if you have to flavor it, that's okay." So we were able to do a little gastronomy at home. Today, she switches between chocolate and vanilla shakes.

For the first few weeks, I was still the skeptical scientist, so I was journaling every day about the food she ate and her pain levels. The poor thing, we badgered her every morning and every night: "What's your pain?"

Over a 20-day period—where we started at a ten out of ten for pain—the numbers slowly went from nine to eight to seven. At the twenty-day mark, Joy reported her pain level at a zero!

I could not believe my eyes—I could actually see her joint swelling reducing. I was also checking the flexibility of her joints. She went from a very stiff ankle to full extension, which was absolutely amazing! Also, the night terrors she had suffered suddenly stopped, so all of us were getting a good night's sleep.

My husband and I are very strong in our faith, and when Joy was dealing with this latest pain crisis, I prayed, "God, make sure we use this one. I'll go through this—I'll do whatever you want— let's use this for something good." So when this answer came to us—an answer we did not expect at all—I was given a chance, as a mom and as a physician, to get the word out about how important and how critical nutrition really is.

After starting the Young Health Shake, I started to ask some of my immunology colleagues, as well as some of my allergy colleagues, about things like the delayed allergy testing Dr. Young had insisted upon, the potential issues created by gluten, and incorporating food and nutrition as a baseline. For the most part, I got the traditional response: "Diet is not that big of a deal–don't worry about it."

I think all of us reach a point where we have to be ready and willing to look outside of the box. Meeting Dr. Young was an eye-opening experience for me, not just as a mom but also as a provider. I learned there are other ways to take care of the body.

Interestingly, not only did my husband and I take care of our child, but then we said, "We have nothing to lose, let's try it, too!" So both of us went through the delayed food testing and started drinking the shake. Now we have a shake every morning and both of us feel better than we've ever felt.

It's nice to know what your body wants, and what it doesn't want. It's also nice to go out to dinner and order what's appropriate and go home and not feel what I call a 'food coma'. It's nice to go to work and not have headaches or feel tired and sluggish throughout the day.

I've been able to translate this nutritional foundation into my office practice. When I see my patients come in and if things don't quite make sense—I call these the patients who 'walk the fine line,' meaning they don't really have a lot of reserve—it's neat to introduce to them something that is outside of the box. Building the foundational blocks of nutrition, making sure they get the proteins and the oil into their bodies, will help their cells function to the best of their ability. In my profession, the end of the line usually results in the operating room. Most people want to do everything they can before they get to that place.

In fact, the shake has been warmly received. I'll start by saying to the parents or my patients, "This may be a little funky." or "This may be a little bit different, but there is something else I can offer you." And every one of them has been very appreciative and very interested to learn. Sometimes we may end up in the operating room, and occasionally we have, but at least we have set the foundation for those children to have a more successful outcome.

The bottom line is that it makes sense—the body needs good things to function. Avoiding the end result of diabetes, cardiovascular disease or arthritis, is a matter of awareness. The body needs basic building blocks to prevent going down that road. So if we can back up a step or two and provide the body with what it needs, those diseases can be reversed or lessened.

Dr. Young:

Once Karin was fully on board with our program and was having success, I was wondering what other physicians had to say when Karin told them what she was doing for Joy.

Karin:

I have to say, the reaction I got from Joy's doctors and still get when I talk about Dr. Young's program, has been mixed. I think there's a portion of physicians out there who *do* want to think outside of the box, especially those I know personally who have seen what we've struggled with as parents. And they're saying that if it's really working and there's scientific evidence behind it, they want to know and want see it! I think we all, as providers, feel like we have some patients we just can't quite figure out, so it's great to have an alternative.

Then there are the more traditional physicians who are comfortable doing what they have been doing and aren't ready to think outside of that box just yet.

Looking back at my time in medical school, I think I have a new perspective to support that nutrition is definitely not emphasized enough. We spend a lot of time in pharmacology and learning how to mask problems and lesson symptoms. I am hopefully though that we are becoming more open-minded about preventive health care.

Dr. Young:

What's really exciting for me in my practice—where I have finally gotten back to getting to the root of the problem and believing you need to lay the foundation—is this: you *can* get people better. My patients don't have to be on twenty or thirty drugs and only have hope to see a less steep decline in quality of life.

As a physician, I asked myself, "Are we here to really get people better or just put them on the protocols?" Once I moved away from those protocols, it's been really amazing.

I love to play tennis in my free time and I can't play as much tennis anymore because there is such a long line of patients waiting to see me. This is happening because people are hearing from their friends and relatives, "I'm getting better!" The calls are coming in with people saying, "Listen, I hear what you did for my neighbor's kid!" That is so satisfying.

That is the reason I wanted to be a doctor in the first place…to make people better!

18. Jane A.

I heard about the Young Health Shake from my dear friend, Karin Hotchkiss, who told me she was having some great success with her daughter, Joy. I thought my 16-year-old daughter, Emily, might be able to benefit from the shake herself. Emily has learning disabilities, along with some communication issues. At a very young age, she was diagnosed with a language delay—which we found out later was apraxia, a speech motor issue— so sometimes it's hard for her to get words out. She knows what she wants to say, but it's hard for her to communicate at times. She will get hung up on words and hung up on what she wants to say.

She was seeing a neurologist—we were actually working with three neurologists until we settled on the one—and it was always my suspicion that she had some nutritional deficiencies and some food sensitivities, particularly to wheat, gluten and dairy. Her skin quality was not good and she just always seemed to be in a fog.

Within the first two weeks of her being on the Young Health shake, she lost between five to seven pounds and she was less swollen all over, especially in her stomach area. Plus, her skin improved, she was more energetic and yes, even her communication ability improved. She seemed to be speaking clearer and her thoughts flowed a lot easier.

The nutritional testing with Dr. Young also proved that my initial instincts were confirmed— those food sensitivities were impacting her nutrition and her overall functioning. What's interesting is that her neurologist was always looking for the anaphylaxis kind of reaction, the breaking out in huge hives kind of reaction. I remember him saying, "She has these mild sensitivities, but don't worry about it. She's fine. It would be a really difficult and restrictive diet to put her on, anyway." And I believed what he had said. But now that we have extracted the wheat, gluten and dairy from her diet, it's like she's come out of the fog.

Overall, Emily just feels better. She recently said to me, "Mom, I don't get headaches anymore." She's so happy that she can simply go into her closest, grab a pair of jeans and fit so nicely into them.

What's also amazing to me is the unsolicited comments we have received about Emily. One day, a good friend said to me, "Wow, Emily's tongue seems to have shrunk and actually fits in her mouth better. She's really speaking clearer." And I know exactly what he is talking about because there were times when I would tell Emily to keep her mouth closed, to keep her tongue inside.

My sister hadn't seen Emily in a while and they spent some time together in our home. When Emily went upstairs to go to bed, my sister said to me, "Wow! There's a huge difference in her communication!"

Also, my oldest daughter is a freshman in college. Recently she came home for the weekend, and I asked her, "Have you noticed anything different about your sister?" And she said, "You know, Mom, it's really interesting that you asked. Emily was telling me a story and it just came out so much smoother, so much easier than it would normally."

I used to give Emily protein and oil in her diet (I used to supplement her with fish oils), and even at a young age, she showed some improvement. However, it wasn't until I learned about the Young Health Shake and how important it is to combine those omega oils with the protein at the same time to get the maximum benefit that I really saw a great improvement in her communication skills.

Since it's possible to use a number of different proteins, Emily is taking the egg white protein because she is sensitive to whey. She has a shake every morning—she loves it and actually looks forward to it because we change it up a little bit. Sometimes it's fruity; sometimes it's banana and chocolate.

My biggest concern with putting her on a very restrictive diet was that she would never feel satiated, but it was a very seamless transition and she has never complained about being hungry.

It is my goal to get everybody in my family on this particular method of protein and nutritional supplements. I had myself tested, and I also drink the protein shake. (I'm just not as a rigorous about it as I am with Emily because I don't have the broad sensitivities that she does.) Within the first three months, I lost five pounds and my digestive issues cleared up, which for me was huge! There is no doubt about it—Dr. Young's program is truly amazing!

19. Christy W.

As a mom of a child with Down Syndrome, I always sensed my now 10-year-old son's body was lacking something, even something minor. I knew it could be fixed—it was just finding what it was that he was missing. Shawn was always sick, and children with Down Syndrome are prone to other conditions. In Shawn's case, it was ear infections, sinus problems and chest congestion, and this told me that something in his immune system was not working properly.

Despite having frequent colds and taking antibiotics for these infections, Shawn has always been a relatively healthy child. We never had any of the heart issues and some of the other more serious illnesses that come with this condition, so we feel very fortunate. Our area of struggle had to do with his ability to learn. We always knew Shawn would be a little bit behind in learning, and I never thought he would be able to write. I just figured that we would have to rely on technology to help him.

Then a special friend of mine introduced me to Dr. Young. As I learned from him, it's really important to start with the foundation—putting the protein and the oil back into the body. Children with Down Syndrome lack amino acids, so we have to add a few things to the shake.

My son takes two shakes a day. I make it with almond milk and chocolate syrup.

Shawn has been taking the shake for a little over a year and he has taken giant steps. His comprehension has multiplied. Before it would take us weeks to do a one-step direction. Now he's doing three-step directions and we can just tell him to do something and he's off doing it. My son can read and write now—he's writing very clearly. He is still struggling with speech, but it's coming.

Also, he's never sick anymore—and he's around sick children all of the time. He's so healthy now because his immune system has been built up. He has not been on one antibiotic in over a year.

Dr. Young also wanted to add glycoproteins (a conjugated protein in which the non-protein is a carbohydrate). At first, I wasn't sure about these proteins until we started giving them to Shawn. It seems that ever since he started taking the glycoproteins, he has made even more leaps and bounds with comprehension, writing and following directions. And he's now taking gymnastics. These are things that we did not think would ever happen for Shawn, but they are happening. It's incredible!

For children like Shawn, it's not so much about making them better but giving them a better quality of life. He's been doing some amazing things, and I think it's because we've been able to research what his body is lacking through blood tests and special urinalysis tests. We've been able to replace the nutrients he's been missing, helping his body to operate and function better.

Here's a funny story. In the beginning, I didn't tell his teachers what we were doing because

I wanted Shawn to be the example. I had no idea if the Young Health Shake was going to work, so I didn't want the teachers to look at us and say, "Let's wait and see if something happens." I wanted Shawn, as always, to be the example of showing how things can work.

The proof is in the pudding, so to speak! One day he sat down with his I.E.P (Individualized Education Plan, a special education plan for each child who has special needs), and his teachers said, "Do we have the right child?" His progress was so dramatic, and it's even more dramatic this year.

The big lesson here is that this Young Health Shake is for everyone—and no matter what condition you may have, it all starts with a foundation, which the shake provides. It's first about getting your body healthy and to get a baseline because anything extra you may need nutritionally has to attach to the proteins.

I think if you do the same thing all the time, you know what your results are going to be. If you try something different, the only thing that can happen is nothing—but you could have the chance of something wonderful coming out of it!

Conclusion

From the beginning of this book to the end, my objective has been to place the way I practice medicine in the context of restoring health to my patients. There is no secret formula. Everything I do comes directly from the practice of medicine, the teaching of medicine, the history of medicine and the latest discoveries in medicine. It has helped that I have a great curiosity and am willing to go the extra mile to find answers.

The biggest problem we now face is that another industry has interfered in the natural course of things. Medicine has become an arm of the pharmaceutical business. Why did this happen? It happened because busy doctors became dependent on the information supplied by the purveyors of drugs. Told by the heads of large practices and insurance companies that "time means money", doctors handed over more and more of their responsibilities to large pharmaceutical companies—the 'big brothers' of the medical world.

Few of us noticed until the practice had become so blatant we were forced to see and admit it. This happened so gradually that people believed they were getting the best treatment medicine had to offer. The problem is, they weren't and they aren't. Patients became a *symptom* needing a *solution*. That solution became a prescription, not an informed application of the doctor's education, history and research of medical knowledge.

The good news? A new group of doctors and patients is now looking with curiosity and excitement at the possibilities of healing and living the optimum life with as few pharmaceutical drugs as possible. The growth in my practice is an indication of the desire by informed patients to be

an important part of their own healing.

Imagine a population of trillions of individuals
living under one roof in a state of perpetual
happiness. Such a community exists. It is called the
healthy human body.
Dr. Bruce Lipton, Ph.D., cell biologist, from
The Biology of Belief

For me, this is an exciting time to be a

physician, as it should be for other healers and

patients. I'm grateful that you came to this book and

look forward to hearing from you as you embark on

your personal journey to complete health.

Appendix

20. Recipes

Young Health Shake Recipes

The Original

> 6-8 oz. Almond Milk/Water/Whole milk
> 1 Scoop Young Health Protein
> 1 tbsp Young Health Flax & Fish Oil Blend
> 10 drops Young Health Balance Drops
> 1 oz Fruit of the Spirit

Vanilla Delight

> 6-8oz. Vanilla Almond Milk
> 1 Scoop Young Health Protein
> 1 tbsp. Young Health Flax & Fish Oil Blend
> 10 drops Young Health Balance Drops
> ½ tsp. Vanilla Extract
> 1 packet of Stevia

Raspberry Cream

> 6-8oz. Vanilla or Original Almond Milk
> 1 Scoop Young Health Protein
> 1 tbsp. Young Health Flax & Fish Oil Blend
> 10 drops Young Health Balance Drops
> 1 cup fresh Raspberries
> 1 tsp. Raspberry sugar free coffee syrup
> ½ teaspoon Vanilla Extract

The Fruit Smoothie

6-8oz. Almond Milk
1 Scoop Young Health Protein
1 tbsp. Young Health Flax & Fish Oil Blend
10 drops Young Health Balance Drops
½ cup frozen blueberries
½ cup frozen raspberries
½ cup crushed ice

Frozen Yogurt Shake

6-8oz. Vanilla Almond Milk
1 Scoop Young Health Protein
1 tbsp. Young Health Flax & Fish Oil Blend
10 drops Young Health Balance Drops
1oz. Fruit of the Spirit
1 cup crushed ice
Small container of low-sugar Yogurt

Chocolate Mocha

6-8oz. Chocolate Almond Milk
1 Scoop Young Health Protein
1 tbsp. Young Health Flax & Fish Oil Blend
10 drops Young Health Balance Drops
1/8th -1/4th teaspoon instant coffee
4-6oz Vanilla low sugar yogurt
½ crushed ice